🪷Poems

From the Passionate Heart

Reflections on Healing and Awakening

Dear Connie,

May blessings,

Poems from the Passionate Heart
Reflections on Healing and Awakening

Holman Health Connections
1917 Rockefeller Ave., Everett, WA 98201 USA
www.holmanhealthconnections.com
Holmanhealth@gmail.com

Softcover Edition ISBN   978-0-9837293-0-3

First Edition 2012

Cover Photo: I took this photo of a False Hellebore while on a hike in Washington's North Cascades, and decided to use it for the cover since it reminded me of opening, awakening, peeling back the layers of our humanness and revealing our biggest, most beautiful and spiritual Self.

I found out later that this plant (Veratrum viride) is an herbaceous perennial belonging to the lily family, and is actually very poisonous! There is a legend that the plant was used by some native tribes to elect a new leader. Each aspiring leader would eat the root, and the last to start vomiting would become the new leader! Another legend claims the plant to be an antidote to madness. May this book help reduce your madness and increase your gladness!

ACKNOWLEDGMENTS

It took a village to help me survive my dark night of the soul, and a community to edit and publish this book. So many people helped me, first, to claw and crawl my way along my inner journey, and secondly, with the specific writing, editing and design of this book.

Let me begin with some of the many people who guided me along my inner journey. Thanks to Susan Picard, my first therapist, and David Calof--hopefully one of my last--as well as all the others in between: Catherine, Robert, Debbie and Mary. Thanks to Anaiis Sales, my hands-on energy healing teacher; Tracy Weber, my main yoga teacher; Jamal Rahman, my teacher of Sufi wisdom; Nancy, my eating disorder 12 step sponsor, Amma, the "Hugging Saint," and Amma Bhagavan for helping me wake up a bit. There are too many others to mention here, but thank you all!

Thank you Mother Earth: the trees, flowers, streams, lakes, bears, frogs, plants, dirt, rocks and countless expressions of life, for nourishing me when I had nowhere else to turn, or when humans scared me too much for me to seek comfort there.

For the specific book help, thanks to all my friends who read and provided feedback: Kaje, Ricky, Donna, Rebecca, Shonagh, Arden, Mari, David, Laura, Tony, Bill, Barb, Stef, Corrina, and Vicki. Thanks to book designer Linda Lapping for her soulful artistry, and Kelley Guiney and Gary Perless for their generous spirit and fine editing. Thank you Shannon and friends at Snohomish Publishing, and Harry and friends at New Leaf Paper, for friendly green printing and publishing.

This book is dedicated to each and every human being, and especially to anyone who has felt and faced the fears, doubts, grief, angst and confusion of being human during these trying and transformative times on planet Earth. May you know your courage, recognize your beauty, and shine bright in the glory and greatness of who you really are.

CONTENTS

INTRODUCTION..9

POEMS:

Birth of an Activist – *March 26, 1991* 11

Dad – *March 16, 1996* 12

Self Hate – *March 20, 1996* 13

Enough! – *March 30, 1997*..14

Food Purist – *September 3, 1997* 15

The Binge – *September 20, 1997* 16

Giving Up? – *November 16, 1997*....................................17

How Low? – *December 1, 1997*..18

What Am I? – *January 8, 1998*...19

Rated R for Rage – *January twenty fucking fifth, 1998* 20

Stuff – *June 13, 1998*..21

Where is God? – *October 12, 1998*.................................22

Universe Within – *November 18, 1998* 23

War Budget Blues – *December 12, 1998*..........................25

Whose Pain? – *December 17, 1998*..................................26

Spirit Unbound – *January 18, 1999*.................................27

Illusion of Separation – *January 20, 1999*.......................28

Eating My Way to God – *January 27, 1999*......................29

Healing Ourselves – *May 3, 1999*....................................32

Hangin' out with Jesus – *June 27, 1999* 34

Unmasked – *November 8, 1999* 35

I am Me – *April 16, 2000*...36

Hopeless – *May 23, 2000*...37

September 11th – *September 12, 2001* 38

Humble Human – *March 17, 2002* 39

I Need to Know – *January 25, 2003* 40

Approval – *February 1, 2003* 41

Courage – *February 3, 2003* 42

Power Never! – *March 1, 2003* 43

Smile, the Warrior's Weapon – *March 12, 2003* 44

Depression's Voice – *June 8, 2003* 45

Male Power – *June 15, 2003* 46

Who You Are – *June 20, 2003* 47

Mind, Be Still – *July 1, 2003* 48

Waiting – *August 12, 2003* 49

River's Flow – *August 14, 2003* 50

Dead End Job – *August 26, 2003* 51

God-Man-Made – *September 21, 2003* 52

Haiku – *October 9, 2003* 53

Unlit – *October 9, 2003* 54

Boxed and Buried – *October 24, 2003* 55

Threshold – *November 15, 2003* 56

Bliss of Denial – *December 25, 2003* 57

Obsessive Healing – *January 25, 2004* 58

April Fool – *April 1, 2004* 59

Feel! – *February 18, 2005* 60

No Worries – *September 1, 2005* 61

Earth Dance – *September 7, 2005* 62

Surrounded Alone – *September 20, 2005* 63

Three Doors – *September 25, 2005* 64

Yoga – *September 25, 2005* 65

The Compassionate Heart – *October 1, 2005* 66

Wonders and Wanders – *December 1, 2005* 67

Acceptance – *January 12, 2006* 68

Heaven or Hell? – *April 30, 2006* 69

Nature's Embrace – *June 1, 2006* 70

Madness – *June 13, 2006* 71

Surrender – *June 21, 2006* 72

Relationship Jitters – *August 1, 2006* 73

Trust – *September 1, 2006* 74

Here Now – *November 12, 2006* 75

Presence – *December 8, 2006* 76

Death be Darned – *March 5, 2008* 77

The Lie of Loneliness – *July 21, 2008* 78

Pain Prayer – *February 7, 2009* 79

How is this Possible? – *February 10, 2009* 80

Overflowing – *February 10, 2009* 81

Open Doors – *February 12, 2009* 82

Valentine's Day – *February 14, 2009* 83

Renunciation – *March 3, 2009* 85

What Would I Do? – *March 15, 2009* 86

Five Again – *March 18, 2009* 87

Anger Again – *March 25, 2009* 88

Consistently Inconsistent – *April 14, 2009* 89

Disaster Denied – *April 18, 2009* 90

The Step – *April 20, 2009* 91

Scorched Earth – *Rainier July 5, 2009* 92

No Ordinary Moments – *July 5, 2009* 93

Frog Feelings – *August 7, 2009* 94

Dance in the Dark – *September 5, 2009* 95

Too Late? – *October 10, 2009* 96

Battle Ready – *October 20, 2009* 97

Cosmic Crayon – *November 1, 2009* 98

What Control? – *December 7, 2009* 99

Fear Not – *December 12, 2009* 100

Breath of the Manta Ray – *December 18, 2009* 101

Life in America – *December 20, 2009* 102

Relationship – *December 20, 2009* 103

The Teacher – *December 22, 2009* 104

Angry-Loving Mother – *December 25, 2009* 105

Awaken! – *December 29, 2009* 106

2010 – *January 1, 2010* 107

Nature Knows – *June 8, 2010* 108

Body Spirit – *November 1, 2010* 109

Catastrophe or Ecstasy? – *November 5, 2010* 110

Resurrection – *December 25, 2010* 111

Courageous Contemplation – *1/1/11* 112

Nature Prayer – *February 2, 2011* 113

Earth Day – *April 22, 2011* 115

Unfiltered Feet – *May 3, 2011* 116

Who I Am – *June 14, 2011* 117

Cedar Wisdom – *June 25, 2011* 118

Be You – *July 11, 2011* 119

Message to the Dark Side – *July 15, 2011* 120

Sacred Masculine – *July 20, 2011* 121

Aging Grace – *July 23, 11* 123

Pain Poems, Passion Poems – *August 1, 2011* 125

INTRODUCTION

These neatly typed verses do not accurately represent my desperate, often teary-eyed words scribbled in various notebooks and journals over the past 20 years. As I scrawled these writings, I assumed they were just for me, some sort of personal raging and purging from a depressed, desperate and delirious man. I believed--or at least hoped--that these were a safe and healthy method of self expression and catharsis.

It was years later that I recognized a part of me that truly wanted to share, to teach, to serve, and I wondered, "Could my rambling expressions and pathetic struggles be of use to someone else? Is my own search part of a bigger story? Is this less about *me* and more about *we*?"

I doubted it, for I have long struggled with self doubt-- even self loathing. So my desperate doodles (I could not call it poetry, which sounded like something important or talented people wrote), like all areas of my life, I deemed wretched and insignificant. Publishing these writings is a significant step outside my comfort zone. Yet my heart called them forth, so here they are.

These writings are arranged in chronological order. In the first draft, I had the poems neatly organized in ten categories, but I soon realized that this is first and foremost autobiographical poetry. By arranging the poems by date, I hope the reader can follow and witness my waves of healing and transformation-- from depression and despair to ever-growing joy and gratitude- -and therefore be motivated for his or her own inner journey. Indeed, you will notice a distinct trend throughout the book, from fear to love.

Be forewarned that some of the earlier writings include some significant gloom, hate, profanity and rage--such was my state of mind. They are more pain than poem. I spent considerable time inside the metaphorical cave--my dark night of the soul- -and emerged with an evolving new, or ancient, world view. Thankfully, there are traces of humor throughout, even amidst the personal chaos and confusion.

As my mind-fog began to lift in my early 50s, I began to see somewhat beyond my own misery and it became clear that I was not the only one in the world struggling with pain, depression, swirling emotions and self hate. I was not alone in my battle to recover from addictions, an eating disorder and sexual abuse. In an interconnected world, one person's struggles, terror and sense of hopelessness are everyone's. One person's joy is everyone's as well.

Within every supposedly lost soul is a fountain of joy and love awaiting discovery and liberation. If just one person reads these words and feels less alone and more alive, then my vulnerability has been worth the risk. In truth, the only thing that can get damaged or diminished is my ego, and this would be good! May these words touch your heart and help awaken your beautiful and most magnificent Self.

Note: I wrote this poem--one of my very first--during the earlier U.S.- Iraq War. I went on to work as a peace activist and human rights educator in Central America for several years.

BIRTH OF AN ACTIVIST   *MARCH 26, 1991*

War is peace, this cause is just.
It is not money and power we lust.

Hussein latest Hitler, aggression must end.
For Kuwait's honor we will defend.

The polls are clear, Americans see,
Push for war; it has to be.

Bombs are fun, just like a game.
They do not hurt, kill or maim.

Cold war's over, peace dividend feigned.
Defense profits must be maintained.

Media's fair, censorship's right.
Revealing more could spoil our fight.

But lies are lies, and some do see,
this is not right, how can it be?

'Cause war's no game, a bomb's not smart,
possesses neither soul nor heart.

And children don't deserve to die,
or lose their mom and wonder why.

So we who have removed our masks,
will wave no flags, we've other tasks.

Note: I returned to the U.S. from Central America in 1996, when my life fell apart. I moved from "outer" activism work to "inner" peace work, and began a dark night of the soul that would last over ten years. Here, I finally grieved my father's death from 30 years earlier.

DAD   *March 1, 1996*

Dad, why didn't you tell me
you were going to die?
Yet another reason to hate you.
You were so angry, abusive, those final years,
drinking, smoking, drugged out,
nasty to us and mom.
Why could you not have been more brave
on your way to the grave?
Dad--and Mom,
you wouldn't share anything,
like the birds and the bees.
You were absent even when you were here.

Dad, if only I had known,
I would have tried harder, been nicer--
I didn't understand the extent of your pain and disease.
"Dad died last night," they told me--just like that.
No goodbye, no resolution, nothing.
Swallowed my feelings yet again.

I'm so sorry, Dad, I could not say goodbye,
tell you I was pissed off, confused,
could not ask you how you felt
or tell you thanks for giving me this life, these lessons,
for providing me with food and shelter,
and brothers and sisters,
for teaching me how to laugh,
for trips to the country--how I loved those trips!
I love you, Dad.
This poem will have to do.

Note: Throughout my 40s, the pain I had unconsciously buried in my body over my lifetime shouted its need to be healed. I reluctantly began to feel old, buried pain, and self hate was my biggest demon.

SELF HATE   *March 20, 1996*

I hate you Roy--that's the truth.
Gotta be fricking perfect?
How arrogant!
You ain't so special!
Who the hell do you think you are?
Jesus? Buddha? God?

Let's be honest--for a change.
You are out of control:
wake up worrying, controlling, planning,
a neurotic piece of shit.
I don't even want to be around you.
That is why people don't truly befriend you;
they sense your crap.

What a God-damned mess you are--
you smell like fear.
I hate you.
Waking up feeling guilty, belly full of food;
don't you ever learn?
I hate you so much.

ENOUGH! *March 30, 1997*

Enough!
You are enough Roy,
and there is enough--do you not see it yet?
There is no scarcity
of anything whatsoever!
Stop worrying, hoarding, planning, controlling . . .
Breathe it in and breathe it out,
an eternal flow.
Jump into the void Roy,
and find it oh so full!

Note: One of the symptoms of my wounds manifested as an eating disorder, with a fixation on a "perfect" raw food diet, with assorted fasts, cleanses and purges.

FOOD PURIST *September 3, 1997*

I have a label: orthorexic.
Food purist.
Aim for perfect health, and crash.
Superior to junk food junkies,
but prisoner to food.
Solitary confinement,
eating alone, disconnected,
food my sole purpose,
(Lord knows my soul purpose).
Afraid to hear the hunger, truly listen.

So much energy invested:
planning, shopping, preparing, sprouting, fermenting,
soaking, blending, smelling, chewing . . .
Obsession without Presence!
Ignoring the feeling which shouts, begs:
connect, reach out, love yourself,
walk, play, surrender.

Just one more meal, alone.
Tomorrow,
I'll listen to the hunger.
Tomorrow.

THE BINGE *September 20, 1997*

Late at night,
hungry again--for something,
wanting to binge.

Out to dinner,
dilemma of what to order--a thousand questions,
then send my plate back.
Poor waitress; I am a pain in the ass.

Back home, straight to the kitchen,
but a breath of power stops me,
a detour to my phone.
12 step sponsor not home,
nor other eating disorder friends,
but the fourth call works,
a voice of sanity and love,
what I cannot find within.

GIVING UP? *November 16, 1997*

I am dead,
certainly not alive.
Obsessed with healing:
time, energy, money
on healers, courses, classes . . .

I am miserable,
forgot how to have fun,
depleted, exhausted, can't sleep,
barely breathing.
So tired of misery
wearing a smiley mask.

What to do?
Travel? Escape?
End my life?
Need I die to be free?

Spirit, I have heard you exist,
hope that you are there,
but I can't find You.
I give up.

How Low? *December 1, 1997*

How low must I fall?
Can't trust myself,
or God--if there is one.
Hating myself, as always.
Where can I turn?

My life is total pain,
physically, mentally, emotionally.
How can one body
hold such a collage of emotions,
easily ignited, sliding me deeper
into my inner swamp
where mud is all I know.

How much does it need to hurt?
How bad does it have to get?
Before I figure this out,
before I surrender,
whatever that means.

WHAT AM I? *January 8, 1998*

Anorexic? Bulimic? Orthorexic?
I don't know.
Addictive personality they say,
certainly obsessive, compulsive.
Just words and labels.
Blame, shame and hate
harder to say or feel.

Yet I can finally say:
eating disorder, I thank you.
You have helped me know
who I am,
lit up my pain,
exposed trauma long buried,
but in such need
of tender attention.

What helps?
Fasting, starvation, rigid control,
self punishment, perfectionism, isolation?
No!

Trusting body, eating when hungry,
following Spirit, connecting with others,
nature, play, expression?
Yes!

Warning: I considered changing the wording on this piece, but need to be honest about the depth of my rage and self hate at the time. This is exactly as I wrote it.

RATED R FOR RAGE   *January twenty fucking fifth, 1998*

Thank you rage
for surfacing,
helping me tell the world,
Fuck you!

God, first of all, great idea,
send us down here to hell on earth.
Nice fucking game!
Watching us go through hell.
Enjoying yourself? You prick!
What's the fucking point?! What?!
Poverty, war, starvation, greed, violence, rape . . .
What's the point?!
Stop the fucking pain!
Stop the madness!
Stop this pressure to be perfect!
I'm GOOD ENOUGH!

Fuck you Mom, fuck you Dad.
Fuck you Catholic Church!
I know, I know--I "created" this.
Well fuck you, too!
I must be a moron, a real masochist
to get myself into this body,
this fucking life.

STUFF *June 13, 1998*

Fear and anger in my face
Still unwilling to go there.
"There"--where pain, perhaps abuse,
lies buried.
Terrifying, but can it hurt me?
It already has!

Am I enraged enough,
depressed enough,
exhausted enough,
bloated enough,
to go there, feel,
be with this stuff?
Every conceivable excuse
to avoid going there.

But step by step
is good enough.

WHERE IS GOD?   *October 12, 1998*

Where is God?
I know, I know--right here,
say the supposedly awakened ones.
Here, everywhere, always.

Well, if you're so almighty,
make yourself clear!
I want answers!
I want my path!
I don't get it!

I just don't know
how to find You,
feel You,
see You,
know You!

UNIVERSE WITHIN   *November 18, 1998*

The world, from the start, has told me what to do.
Taught me how to look outside myself for clues.

From that first day, forty years ago,
greeted with a slap, and a tug on the toe.

Needles and vaccines--circumcision too!
Needless part, removal is the thing to do.

"Ouch ouch," I cried! "Are you quite certain?"
"Trust us, trust us, you're not really hurtin'!"

Have a plastic bottle, no breast do you need.
Bonding's unimportant, you only need a feed.

But something feels funny, where's the loving touch?
Don't be greedy, you're asking way too much.

So off to Catholic school, Sister Mary who?
Sunday service in that rock hard pew.

Do this, don't do that, don't dare make a fuss.
Behave--you sinner. Hey, was that a cuss!

But wait, is it true that God's so judgmental?
I've given up on heaven, God's too temperamental.

I need to talk, express and be heard,
sing and play, not treated like a turd.

I know, I know, born with original sin.
Bad from the start, no chance in hell to win.

Still I graduated, did my very best,
to avoid being punished, passed every test.

Then I tried to do, like all who search for joy,
bought every material good, each consumer toy.

The food I was fed, and later fed myself,
from the market chain--crap on every shelf.

Made me moody and gave me diarrhea.
People call it food; they have no idea.

Still had no clue, of who I really was.
Found beer and booze, to help me get a buzz.

I saw the commercials: beer makes people happy,
until the mornings, I'd wake up feeling crappy.

Drugs, I knew, would solve my woes,
but alas, I only reached the lowest of lows.

Which is where, perhaps, I needed to be,
before I learned to shift the search inside of me.

Finally, thank God, got past the doubt,
to find within, what I thought I was without.

Wisdom and joy, long buried and ignored,
no longer rotten, beauty at the core!

So read books, go to school, follow every guru,
until you find the Universe, awaiting right inside you.

Note: Our annual defense budget and supplementary war spending has more than doubled in today's dollars since I wrote this in 1998. Our 2011 defense budget was about $700 billion dollars, not including discretionary spending and other wars. This represents nearly half of the world's total military spending.

WAR BUDGET BLUES   *December 12, 1998*

Four hundred billion dollars, each and every year
keeps the bad guys from getting too near.

Over 30 billion, every 30 days,
keeps us safe, let me count the ways.

Eight billion dollars, just this very week,
makin' damn sure we don't appear weak.

More than a billion, we will spend today,
big bucks for bombs, our schools in decay.

Fifty million dollars, in this very hour,
strange world this is, where weapons equal power.

Half a million bucks, each and every minute,
to me a wicked waste, now matter how they spin it.

Ten thousand dollars, every second spent
all on war, our fear evident.

WHOSE PAIN?   *Dec 17, 1998*

What do I do,
while we do it again?
We, the world leader
in possession, sales and use
of weapons of mass destruction,
today, this minute, live on TV
using weapons of mass destruction
to bomb Iraq, in case they have
weapons of mass destruction.

What is the source of my angst and tears?
Do I feel Iraqi pain?
Anger at my country or leaders?
Sadness at our primitive behavior?

Or is this just a reflection,
of my inner turmoil,
my own pain triggered?

I only know
that I must cry.

Note: I wrote these words on MLK Jr's birthday, in 1999, and read it to the "lifer" prisoners at the Correctional Complex in Monroe Washington.

SPIRIT UNBOUND *January 18, 1999*

You are all free--can you not see?
Though it may seem untrue, we are all truly free.

As Gandhi has said, and Thoreau I have read,
a soul one cannot imprison, a spirit is never dead.

Words, I first thought, many have taught
to falsely raise hope, where there be naught.

For sure as the night removes the light,
I'm victim without power, no might and no rights.

Yes, if this you believe, yourself you deceive.
For from this prison, this moment, your spirit can leave.

Your spirit is not tied to a body denied.
Your soul lives forever when the body has died.

Of course this does not say, we accept this way,
of choosing ever more walls, locking ourselves away.

Power is not found where fear and judgment resound.
There are no limits to a spirit unbound.

Can you not see, that those who hold the key,
are not guards, guns and gates, but each of us, you and me.

ILLUSION OF SEPARATION   *January 20, 1999*

Where have we failed?
So many jailed.
A people imprisoned,
freedom derailed.

Separation, from here it stems.
It's not us, it's them.
But separation is an illusion.
Here is the gem:

Those who we fear,
offer a bright, shiny mirror,
to see that part of ourselves
we avoid, though so near.

For I say to you,
what to others we do,
we do to ourselves.
Here is the clue:

We are all one;
separate is no one.
When I see me in you,
freedom is won.

Note: This story is partly fiction, but it captures the essence of my eating and fasting adventure, and giving my power away to a food guru.

EATING MY WAY TO GOD   *January 27, 1999*

Sitting at the juice bar, one fine sunny day,
met a cool guy--called himself Ray.
We got to talking about food and health and stuff.
He said he liked his "bounty in the rough."
Feeling ignorant, I asked, "What do you mean?"
as I noticed, he appeared quite strong and lean.
"Raw food," he said, "is the only way to go."
I had to admit, he had quite a glow,
bright clear eyes--a look of confidence.
"Cooked food is dead," he said, "It's just common sense;
kills the life force, and every living enzyme.
Wish we could talk more," he said, "but I'm all out of time."

So off he went, but left me quite certain,
my diet, I now knew, was causin' all my hurtin.'
So raw I went, filled my home with sprouts and fruits,
grabbed the tofu, rice, and beans, gave it all the boot.
Felt strong, light and clear, oh so fast.
I was committed--goodbye poisons of the past!
Got so excited, told everyone I knew:
"I've found the key to happiness--you can do it too!"
They looked at me quite strangely, but what did they know?
So full of toxins, their brains were kinda slow,
to all that junk food, they couldn't say no,
left their colons hangin' heavy and low.

Several months later, lucky my fate,
ran into Ray again, helped me validate,
how righteous I was on this path of mine.
Ray himself was fasting, now on day nine.
"Raw food is key," he said, "but hardly enough;

we need to fast, to clean out all the stuff."
So home I went, tossed out all my food,
imagining my intestines becoming unglued.
Water-only fast, ignoring friends' weird looks,
"Fasting Can Save your Life"--showed 'em Shelton's book.
They still didn't get it, so I offered a clue:
"Jesus and Gandhi did it; they knew what to do!"
Two weeks later, and ten pounds lighter,
so cleansed I glowed, eyes never brighter.

But months later, and my vibrancy receded,
cravings of the past, crying to be heeded.
Feeling disappointed, not yet quite pure.
Was this the path? No longer was I sure.
I needed support, and this was my lucky day,
for who do I run into, but my good friend Ray!
Helped me confirm, "Just a healing crisis," he said,
but then I noticed, his eyes a bit red.
"What's up Ray?" I asked, "*You* couldn't be sick?"
"I'm fine, just fine," he answered real quick.
"Silly thought," I laughed, "of course you're okay."
"Just detoxing," he mumbled, and quickly walked away.

One year later, was when I hit the wall.
Weak or not, I had to heed the call.
Dying for something cooked--Mexican sounds terrific,
or Thai or Chinese--but would it make me sick?
"I don't care," I cried, "gotta have it now,
baked, fried or barbecued, I don't care how."
Made sure no one saw me, looked up and down the street,
entered a buffet, sign said, "All You Can Eat!"
Didn't give doubt a chance, didn't hesitate,
right to the food, filled a heaping, steamy plate.
What remained of guilt receded with that first bite,
how delicious--tasted oh so right!

Then, I couldn't believe it, at first he looked away,
but eating at the very next table, was my good friend Ray!
Our eyes met--a moment of shame.
I even felt pissed off--him I wanted to blame.
Then a huge smile slowly lit his face,
I felt all my anger disappear without a trace.
We stared in silence, giddy with grace.
"Beat ya for seconds," I cried; we grabbed our plates in a race.
We ran like children who never knew of guilt,
beautiful sculpted delicacies on each plate we built.
We sat down together, Ray said, "You know,
raw food's great, but I hadda say, Whoa!
When we get so focused on what we gotta eat,
friends, family and fun take a back seat."
The waitress came by; I ordered a round of beers.
"I'm so tired," I said, "of living life in fear.
I got so thin and yin, haven't had sex in years!"
We laughed so hard, our eyes filled with tears.
"We got too rigid," said Ray, "our lives trying to perfect,
as if we joined some zealots in some cult or crazy sect.
Moderation, balance, perhaps this is the key."
"Except for today," I said, "more food and beer for me!"
No more depriving my beautiful bod.
Who says we can't eat our way to God?

HEALING OURSELVES *May 3, 1999*

I look all around; confusion surrounds
a planet in pain, freedom locked and bound.
So I tried, oh how I tried,
to heal this world, but my hands felt tied.
With ever more war, I fell knees to the floor,
"Where can I start? I need to do more."

It took quite awhile; I felt impatient and riled.
Then a message came clear: *Why not start with a smile?*
"For a smile you call!? Of all the gall!
A world at war, and a smile's gonna change it all!?"
The response came joyously, *No, not just a smile, you see.*
It all starts with you; the smile and joy you must be.
"But how can I "be" joy? I feel so annoyed.
I have so much to do--give me a plan to deploy."

Then put yourself to this test, why not "do" a bit less?
Take a look at yourself, if truly peace is your quest.
For it all starts within. Heal yourself to begin.
Or not, it's your choice. There's no such thing as sin.

"Well, surely now you jest. Don't blame me for this mess.
I'm a peaceworker you know, always done my best."
No blame do I lay; you asked so I say.
Can you bring peace to the planet,
when fear and hate guide your way?

"Are you some sort of nut!?
There's no fear or hate in this gut!
Although, I admit, in this very moment,
I'd like to kick your butt!"

Oh, that's right, forgive my oversight.
You're a peacemaker, of course. No need to fight.

But you might keep in mind, we are all one of a kind.
It is not we versus they, we are one, you will find.
And if peace is your goal, then let this be your role:
let go of the dark, and let light fill your soul.

HANGIN' OUT WITH JESUS   *June 27, 1999*

*Note: Special thanks to the anonymous author of a similar poem I read
at Kuan Yin Tea House in Seattle, titled, "I Meet the Buddha."*

All across the land I searched far and wide,
to meet this wise man Jesus, I would not be denied.
Patience paid off one day, in the garden he was found,
an aura of peace all 'round him, could be heard not a sound.

"Jesus, please help me, it is enlightenment I seek."
He turned my way gently, though anything but meek.
"Jesus, tell me, how can I be perfect like you?"
"Beats me," he replied, "I haven't got a clue."
"Ah, humor," I said, "to lighten my quest!
But seriously, I want perfection, nothing less."
"Let's enjoy the garden," he said, and sat beneath a tree.
"Sounds great," I said, knowing soon I would see.

Hangin' out with Jesus, just my lucky day!
But my patience waned, as I awaited what he'd say.
A breeze picked up, my mind raced.
A chance to learn from Jesus, I did not want to waste.
Soon my butt grew oh so sore,
then I heard from Jesus, a not-so-gentle snore.
Man, this guy's a bloody bore--
I can't take this, not a second more!
"Jesus Christ, never mind, I'll do it my way!"
"Right on dude," he smiled, and rolled the other way.

UNMASKED *November 8, 1999*

How hard, at first, to see,
what I thought myself to be:
weathered, fixed, permanent,
could this mask be all of me?

Alas there is beneath it,
a gentle baby boy,
who learned to survive
by hiding pain and joy.

Mask I thank you so,
what a deed you've done.
You've danced, grinned and followed
the needs of everyone.

Thus, the thought of life alone,
a certain death I fear,
should someone get a glimpse
of my power, hate or tears.

A last horrific pause.
Can I really put you down?
Can I stop being
the puppet and the clown?

This is the day,
the dawn's light reveals,
the man behind the shield,
risking being real.

I AM ME *April 16, 2000*

Alas, now I see
to be truly free
I just be me.
Wheeee!

HOPELESS *May 23, 2000*

Sometimes, like today,
life is impossible.
How can so much pain,
ancient emotions, raw feelings
be stuffed
into such a tiny body?
Do they never end?

SEPTEMBER 11TH *September 12, 2001*

I am the Earth, shaken to the core,
illuminating, cleansing, what has been ignored.

I am the office worker, engulfed in the flame,
and I am the fire, my own life I claim.

I am the Pentagon, war is my job,
preparing for enemies, today, I just sob.

I am the President, struggling for words,
to calm a nation, of my crime absurd.

Yes, I am the terrorist, seething with hate,
proud of mass murder, is this evil innate?

I'm an American, searching outside for answers,
hoping revenge will take out the cancer.

I'm a peace activist, no eye for an eye,
fighting against war, my own rage denied.

The only war that I can win
is through the path that leads within.

For I am God, connected to all,
allowing my lessons, can I hear my own call?

I am love, yet I have hate.
I will not blame others, for what I create.

HUMBLE HUMAN *March 17, 2002*

I am simply human
imperfect like the rest,
releasing the deadly notion
that I have to be the best.

I NEED TO KNOW *January 25, 2003*

Could it be I'm not crazy?
Might there be an explanation
for my constant search for sanity,
new locations, occupations.

Must be a reason
my life's a stinking mess.
What I don't remember
is abuse, nothing less.

What stirs in my gut
like a growling, seething ball?
Threatening its rage,
leaky, porous walls.

Memory you are smart,
choosing what to keep.
But please, I have to know,
I really need some sleep.

APPROVAL *February 1, 2003*

Who writes this poem--
Me, or my fearful ego?

For whom do I write--
for me, for you or for You?

For whom do I live--
For me, for you or for We?
Your approval, your love.

I'm so confused.
I'm so afraid.
I'm so human.
And hopefully more.

COURAGE   *February 3, 2003*

The only thing that scares me
more than remembering the madness
is not.

The only thing that frightens me
more than feeling the pain
is staying numb.

The only thing that panics me
more than the light
is being stuck in the dark.

The only thing that terrifies me
more than opening to heaven
is staying locked in hell.

POWER NEVER! *March 1, 2003*

Power, I seek you not.
Never!
Away, be gone, let me be.

Power: painful and punishing,
I have seen your ugly face,
feared your awful wrath,
tasted your soap and felt your belt,
stung by both sides of your Catholic hand.
Oh, I know you well.

I'm no fool--I've made my choice.
Withered, contracted, silenced, afraid,
but better than you!
Never an evil deed, or anger leak,
safe, hidden, harmless,
as a hand grenade.

SMILE, THE WARRIOR'S WEAPON *March 12, 2003*

A smile, the warrior's weapon.
Change the world, heal the Earth,
simple, easy.

Notice the fear, and smile.
Feel the hate, and be still,
knowing who you are.
Fight for peace, gently,
one breath at a time.
Be an activist, quietly march,
as you see yourself in the enemy you imagine,
and again, smile.
Observe your mistakes, born of ignorance and innocence,
and laugh aloud--ha!

Know that your smile
is the smile that ends all war.
Your genuine smile, not a fearful, frozen phony.
Your beautiful, simple smile,
which has crossed the courageous current from the heart,
more potent than preaching,
more enlightening than the wordy book.

Listen to the music, and smile.
Feel the sun or rain, and smile.
Taste the food of the Earth, and smile.
Know yourself, and smile.
For your smile is God's smile.

Each day, liberate a hundred hungry hearts
with your smile.

DEPRESSION'S VOICE *June 8, 2003*

I'm "officially" depressed.
Therapist suggests anti-depressants,
but am I "against" depression?

Do I need medication, or meditation
to decompress my emotional space?
Pop the lid of some pills,
or remove the suffocating blanket
smothering my life-force and creativity?

Is depression not
just expression unsung,
energy repressed, feelings compressed,
beneath the tears of terror,
behind the damned river of rage.

What if the solution were simply this:
cry and sing and dance and play.
Depression's expression.

MALE POWER *June 15, 2003*

What would it be like, to be a real man?
My body is confused, doesn't understand.

Why, why, your approval I so need,
before I consider every act or deed?

And what is this thing between my legs?
Can I accept it, or forgiveness must I beg?

It's not some ugly, outdated decoration,
more than just a tool for urination.

And what's with this, turning cheek and being meek?
Don't tell me Jesus was wimpy and weak.

Yet force ain't cool, gung ho like GI Joe.
A world out of balance, all push and no flow.

No, I don't support the latest ghastly war.
Yet I'm unafraid to power up and roar.

Leave the head, follow heart and be real.
Connect and learn, how to feel and heal,

Celebrating healthy femininity.
Demonstrating sacred masculinity.

No more war, rage or bitter blame.
Enough of hating self, sin and toxic shame.

We men are not some primitive mistake.
Let's power up, for God's and all our sake.

WHO YOU ARE *June 20, 2003*

Oh my beloved,
There is no need to look
outside yourself
for joy,
for love,
for God.

For you *are*
joy,
love,
God.

MIND, BE STILL *July 1, 2003*

Ah, busy mind
working hand in hand
with an eager ego.
Another clever plan.

We'll be happy when . . .
fill in the blank.
Distracts me so,
from ever feeling thanks.

Mind, do you not see
control is your name?
Or do I expect too much,
since survival is your game.

So, it's up to me
to take the driver's seat.
Be calm, my frenzied friend.
The present is complete.

WAITING   *August 12, 2003*

Waiting, waiting, waiting . . .
For what?
Must be something I lack,
something to bring me joy or peace.
But from where, whom, what?

Waiting feels like resistance to reality,
denial of what is,
a state of anticipation or expectation.

Is it possible to unwait,
wait no more?
To be here, now, present?
Releasing the sharp edge that cuts and controls.
What would this feel like?
What if this moment is complete?

I've been waiting
for what is already here.
I've been searching
for what I already have.
I've been seeking
who I already am.

RIVER'S FLOW *August 14, 2003*

How does the river flow?
Does it judge the occasional obstruction?
Curse the beaver and inevitable logjam?
Fight, resist, struggle?

Or shift, change course, find a new way,
focused, knowing its path
is its own, unique to itself,
unlike other creeks and streams,
some hurried, some calm,
some frigid, some tepid,
some clear, others muddied,
but all flowing
back to the same destination,
unto itself.

Note: For many years, I worked jobs I hated, too afraid to make a change. This is about a job I had in sales for seven years; the last three felt like hell.

DEAD END JOB *August 26, 2003*

Here I stand, unaware,
blank, empty stare.
Suffocated, stifled.
How much more can I bear?

They say we must feed our soul.
Focus on dreams and goals,
or it will eat you from within.
A passionless life takes its toll.

Reacting to fuzzy faces with a forced smile.
Any customer question gets me riled.
Then shame for not being nice.
Thinly masked hate, denial.

What makes me so afraid?
All my dreams aside are laid.
Just how long will I wait?
Until all my visions fade?

GOD-MAN-MADE   *September 21, 2003*

It's all nature.
It's all God.
Everything is natural,
though it may sound odd.

The rock and oak,
salmon and bear.
Cars and roads,
computers and chairs.

Meadow's clear stream,
old growth stand.
Polluted pond,
clear cut land.

But shhhh, be still.
How do you *feel?*
Where is the magic?
What balances and heals?

Careful what we create.
Does it help or harm?
Widen a child's smile,
or trigger inner alarm?

Haiku *October 9, 2003*

This, my first haiku
a simple five-seven-five
How I hate rules.

UNLIT *October 9, 2003*

Lighthouse extinguished.
Illuminates no one's way.
Unseen, does not see.

BOXED AND BURIED *October 24, 2003*

We bodies, you know,
get no respect.
Spirit gets the glamour,
we the neglect.

Cut down trees,
whose own bodies create,
my eternal prison--
overpriced crate.

And how 'bout the Earth
that nourished, help me grow?
It's my turn to share,
as the cycle should go.

But alas, this horrid trick,
inglorious conclusion.
Trapped and wrapped uptight,
eternal seclusion.

Can't feed the animals,
on this Earth I so love,
if sealed and preserved,
in a lonely coffin shoved.

Let my cry now be heard,
while my body has a voice.
Feed me to the Earth--
it's my body and my choice.

THRESHOLD   *November 15, 2003*

I see the threshold
upon which I stand.
Here: despair, terror,
allergies and eating disorder.

I feel where this can go:
chronic fatigue, deepening depression, suicide.

I also see something distant and dreamy,
which presently feels impossible:
eating without distress, consistent energy,
alive, grounded, vibrant,
connected in community,
on a path of passion,
maybe even teaching!

Which will it be?
Is it really up to me?

BLISS OF DENIAL   *December 25, 2003*

Consciousness causes pain.
The depth of one's suffering
matches the level of awareness.

Watch TV, and numb.
Overeat, and numb.
Have a drink, and numb.
Pop a pill, and numb.

But numb is not dumb,
avoiding pain seems smart,
at least for today.
But ah, tomorrow . . .

Consciousness requires courage.
Reality invites responsibility.
Feelings can be fierce,
but alive, awake, aware:
the hero's choice.

OBSESSIVE HEALING *January 25, 2004*

I'm so smart, I'm way cool.
Spiritually superior to all you fools.

I know most everything on this life's mission,
but am still quite humble, and willing to listen.
What the heck, I'll try fasting and raw food.
Down to 99 pounds, self-righteous, skinny dude.

Meditation mellows me, way grounded guy,
for an hour a day, the other twenty-three I fly!
Hands on healing is next on the list,
but what's with this fear, contracted like a fist.

Okay, all right, so I need some more work.
I'll dig deep within, see what demons lurk.
I'll train as a psychic, see and heal my pain,
but lost in a cult, not feeling all that sane.

Cranial sacral, acupuncture, rolfing, chiropractic,
shamanic journey, retrieve my soul, a zillion costly tactics.
12 step, 2 step, yoga, tai chi,
Sufi dancing for world peace, soberly sipping tea.

Still, I hate everyone, especially myself,
despite the thousand self help books on my shelf.
Raging and exhausted, where next can I turn?
Why am I still imperfect, what more do I need learn?

Maybe I'll just rest a sec, have a bit of fun,
wait for enlightenment, while soaking up some sun.
Ahhh, how delicious, and surprisingly odd.
The less I search and struggle, the closer I feel to God!

APRIL FOOL   *April 1, 2004*

Angry, yet again.
Is fury forever?
Is therapy endless?
What am I pissed about?
Nothing inspires me--nothing.
50-year-old loser: no home, no wife, no life.
Hopeless, helpless,
inconsistent, incompetent.
Victim--but of who, what?
My own inability or unwillingness to live.

What would I do,
if I were a real man?
How would I feel
if I weren't so flawed?
I'm so tired of being me,
or whoever this is.

FEEL! *February 18, 2005*

I FEEL!
What a joy!
Countless years of desperate,
exhausted attempts at containment
and inevitable toxic leaks.
What relief!

Feeling pain isn't fun,
but even if our past was insane,
what is more insane than burying it
or wrapping it up
and carrying it with us?
Let go!

Sane is sensing, allowing, relating, listening
to our worn down but beloved body,
always present and precious.
Feel!

Follow the feelings
to freedom.

No Worries   *September 1, 2005*

Look back
with eyes from beyond
and ask yourself:

Has worry ever taken you
one step closer
to God?

EARTH DANCE   *September 7, 2005*

Dance light through your eye.
Prance prana up the spine.
Sing hymns from the heart.
Breathe chi earth to feet.

The entire Universe
is listening, playing
as your audience
and orchestra.

SURROUNDED ALONE *September 20, 2005*

Look for the lie
lurking beneath your loneliness.
A relationship can never end,
and you cannot be alone
any more than you can stroll through a forest
unheard, unseen,
by yourself.
Feel your Companions!
Feel your Self!
Everywhere!

THREE DOORS *September 25, 2005*

Around the pain,
or into the pain?

Careful!
The easy, first choice leads to momentary relief,
followed by familiar frustrations,
death and decay.

The second choice enmeshes us,
wallowing in pitiful and everlasting
emotional angst, pity, pain.

But a third door invites us
through and beyond the den of demons,
the terrain of transformation,
alchemical paradise,
where angels sing
praises to your power.

YOGA *September 25, 2005*

Asana,
let the dance begin.
Beloved body,
dancing to Earth's vibration.

Pranayama,
breath of the Divine.
Purring songs to the shadows.
Life force to each limb's leaf.

Dhyana,
the frantic search subsides.
With a knowing smile,
sense the one world within.

Samadhi,
beyond the veil,
illusion be gone.
Joy beyond joy,
holiest of holy.

Yoga is an invitation
back to the body,
back to the present,
back home.
Namaste.

THE COMPASSIONATE HEART *October 1, 2005*

That which you deny
deadens and destroys.
What you resist
remains, renews.
What you hate
you recreate.
What you fear
you draw near.
That which you judge
you are, have been, or will become.

But what you see clear
offers a mirror.
What you allow, breathe into
softens, shifts--in its own time.
What you hold gently
in your heart
heals.

Wonder within?
Or wander the world?
Inner journey,
or outer journey?
Which is the wiser path to find oneself?

Fret not, my friend.
With a willing heart
and open eye,
every path purifies.
All roads intersect
and self reflect.
Nowhere
will you not be found.

ACCEPTANCE *January 12, 2006*

Your strength
is in your willingness
to be weak.

Your power
is in your courage
to feel.

Your joy
is in your presence
with despair.

Your divinity
is in your acceptance
of your humanity.

Heaven or Hell? *April 30, 2006*

If I give up the fight
what more could I write?
Does poetry not require
drama, conflict and fright?

Perhaps, like Rumi,
rather than gloomy,
I could sing my praise,
more bloomy than doomy!

But again doubt returns
with cautious concerns.
What if I brighten too soon?
Joy overturned.

I know caution well,
fear's familiar smell.
So, what the hell--
I'll give heaven a spell!

NATURE'S EMBRACE   *June 1, 2006*

Have you ever
brushed your cheek lightly
on soft cedar bark?
Or felt grass and twigs,
through undefended feet?

Have you ever
thanked your beating heart
for climbing mountain's trail?
Felt cells sing when plunging body
into clear, alpine lake?
Or lay sun-soaked flesh
on cool forest floor?

Have you danced naked
in rainforest mist,
absorbed nature's ionic prana
of wilderness waterfall?

Have you ever . . .
let nostrils and senses take you
info forest's dimming light
where eyes cannot reach?
Or matched the rhythm of your heart
to singing stream's song?

And have you recognized in all of this,
your own beloved beauty,
your own powerful presence,
your own sacred Self?

MADNESS *June 13, 2006*

There, in that look of approval--
this is what I seek!
Or perhaps here,
in the heady realm of knowledge
and institutional intelligence.
But it does not last.

Fame, then, surely
will satisfy my egoic thirst,
or wealth will curtail my frantic search.
Wrong again--is this world empty?

How can You be so close,
and I remain so hungry and lost?
Are you so bright,
that I am blind?

The wise ones say,
"Be still and know I am God,"
as I pace, desperate and depressed.

If this be so, that I am God,
then God is an anxious madman!
Or perhaps mad is this man
who has not found You.

SURRENDER   *June 21, 2006*

Terrifying to me, this little egoist me,
the threat of annihilation,
dissolving my drop of distinction
into the ocean of Absolute,
inglorious surrender of all I have carefully created
into death and destruction.

Perhaps, rather than merge with the Almighty,
let the Almighty emerge
from the depths of my heart.

Ahh, mind and intellect,
you seek control and understanding.
Relax and breathe.
Trust and melt
into waves of the One,
arms of the Beloved.
Lose self.
Find Self.

Ah, delightful demons,
once again I am impressed,
shaking my head in awe
at your clever creativity,
mind's many methods
of diverting me from pain.

"Trust me--this way,"
back to solitary confinement,
leaving me safely miserable,
afraid of the very connection I need
to heal, love, be loved.

Though relationship leads into the heart of hell,
it perturbs the betrayals and bitterness,
enlightens the darkness,
and stirs the soul
into life worth living.

TRUST *September 1, 2006*

Crumble your walls.
Break down your borders.
Disable alarms.
Tear down your fences.
Unlatch your doors.

I am friendly.
Let Me in.
Let your Self out.

HERE NOW   *November 12, 2006*

Darkness,
depression
despair.

Where is the light?
the joy?
the hope?

Within the darkness.
Beneath the depression.
In the heart of despair.

PRESENCE *December 8, 2006*

The one who sits with fear
is unafraid.
The presence with pain
does not suffer.
The awareness of depression
cannot be repressed.
The observer of insanity
is not crazed.
The witness of anger
holds no bitterness.
The silence surrounding confusion
is quietly clear.
The light within the dark
sees.
The love that lives in the heart of hate
heals.

Note: I wrote this poem the day after my Mother's death.

DEATH BE DARNED   *March 5, 2008*

Death be darned,
evil and inevitable.
No one escapes it.
Everyone survives it.

Death is birth,
transition and doorway.
Dark cannot exist without light.
Tunnels have two round doors.

When I pass through,
feel, grieve, spend yourself--
yet delay not the celebration!
Rejoice, rebirth, renew,
recycle my well-worn body.
Burn it, bury it, feed it to the wolves,
for fire, dirt and teeth affect me not.

Listen, listen . . .
words from the woods,
whispers in the wind,
above, below, within you.
I am with you
always . . .

THE LIE OF LONELINESS *July 21, 2008*

Such a lie, this loneliness.
Look around!
Though it may not appear,
as in a mirror,
furred, feathered, scaled, branched,
green, gray, wet, or brittle,
your one and only Friend,
wearing countless cloaks.

Note: This poem refers mainly to an "accident," when my car was hit by a semi truck on a Washington freeway in 2002, causing me a career change and years of pain, medical expenses, drama and fuel for my inner victim!

PAIN PRAYER *February 7, 2009*

Teacher,
I bow to you,
honor, praise you.
For you have shoved me, spun me,
stopped me in my tracks,
shouted: this is your new path!

You have changed my life and career,
forced me to face lifetimes
of helpless and powerless patterns,
urged me to raise my voice,
taught me self care and compassion,
invited me to seek my soul,
and treasure my body.

Together, we have spent
countless demanding days
and sleepless nights.
I have cursed you and closed,
embraced you and opened.

As I tell my story,
some call me unfortunate victim
and you an ugly and godless mistake.
How I love to agree!

But today,
I, the brave and blessed one,
call you friend.

How is this Possible? *February 10, 2009*

Careful here, caution;
ego can swell with this.
But I must ask, in awe, in all humility;
how is it that I have come to teach?

How has this insignificant, disempowered
pathetic wanderer come to share
this most profound and healing
science and art of yoga?

It is You who helped me
move one step,
change one thought,
feel one feeling,
take one breath,
nervously, desperately,
adjusting to the vibration
of your beloved breath.

OVERFLOWING   *February 10, 2009*

Half empty or half full?
A worthy question.

The wise one sees
the ocean in every drop.

Come plunge and bathe
in the ecstatic waters,
Divine's eternal waterfall.

OPEN DOORS *February 12, 2009*

It is beyond me
what stirs these changes,
but one by one,
my prayers are being answered.

Open a window of faith
in the castle of doubt.
Move one step
through the quagmire of fear.
Allow just a crack
in the impenetrable heart.
Spirit enters from every door.

Spend less time looking back at closed doors
and leap through the open one!

VALENTINE'S DAY   *February 14, 2009*

Another year, another failed relationship.
Will I ever find my true love?

Lay down your violin!

Every relationship is a gift, lesson, and blessing,
a discovery, a willingness to engage
in humanity's greatest and most treacherous challenge:
courageously connecting with other human beings.
Longevity cannot be the measure of each holy encounter--
all human experiences temporary.

Moreover, here you are engaged
in a most magnificent and glorious,
lifelong, committed relationship
with yourself!
Body, mind and spirit--seemingly impossible task!

Relentless and unshakeable,
you have studied, sought, searched,
begged, prayed and pleaded
to know thyself in every uncomfortable and inglorious detail.
You have sunk into your shadows, cried in the dark,
become intimate with your fear and shame,
befriended your demons,
outlasted and redefined
your tragedies and traumas.

You have detested yourself,
yet shown up with flowers.
You have danced openly into the light,
breathed life into your body,
stilled your manic mind, liberated your spirit
and become your most trusted, beloved ally.

And we have yet to mention,
the relationship you have cultivated
with the One who moves this pen.

Do not speak to me of failed relationships, my friend.
This 53 year commitment is a lesson in love,
a mastery and monument to your everlasting journey,
only to discover this:
There is no one else to relate to!
Only seeing and being
the one true love.

RENUNCIATION *March 3, 2009*

The true renunciate
is not the one
who abandons earthly luxuries,
trading temporary treasures
for unspeakable everlasting illumination.

The genuine, if foolish, being
forsakes ecstatic bliss
for momentary materialism
and plastic pleasures.
How brave this explorer!

WHAT WOULD I DO?   *MARCH 15, 2009*

What would I give
for a date with the Divine?
What am I willing to do, or undo
for the grace of your embrace?

Would I surrender addictions to worry, fear and ego?
Would I refrain from judgment and envy?
Would I see myself in the prisoner or politician?
Would I befriend my neighbor,
or feed the poor, honor the least amongst us?
Would I release control and mistrust?
Would I leave a moment of space unfilled,
still my mind, listen, welcome You?

Wise one, show me, teach me,
empower me, have mercy on me.
Reveal my smallness and bigness,
so that I may help light up our world.

FIVE AGAIN *March 18, 2009*

Five years old--again!?
Will I ever grow up?

Only when each and every sensation and wound
has been welcomed,
every frozen feeling
set in the sun of acceptance,
each disconnected, disassociated aspect of the self,
invited home,
embraced and integrated,
each moment of shame,
nourished with tender understanding.

Nothing stays lost forever;
everything is essential.
Here, now, made whole
with bold, compassionate presence
and grace.

ANGER AGAIN   *March 25, 2009*

Anger? You again?!
Am I not done with you?
Layer upon layer.
Is there no end?

Once again, I struggle to take a breath,
begrudgingly lay ego and judgment aside
so I can greet you properly,
see what gifts you bring.

And there, beneath your thorny crust,
within your fearful underbelly,
are the pearls of pain,
followed by torrents of tears,
the tender, delightful release.
Peace and awe.

Anger, old friend,
You are always welcome here.

CONSISTENTLY INCONSISTENT   *April 14, 2009*

Writing about green living
on my plastic computer.

Loving nature,
driving to the trailhead.

Teaching my students independence,
but please approve of me,
and keep coming to my class!

Preaching about presence,
reading while I eat.

Never ever rude or angry,
except with those who can't see it.

Evolved and enlightened,
unless in relationship.

I am an imperfect human
and a perfect contradiction.

DISASTER DENIED *April 18, 2009*

I awaken, tense and terrified--
a normal day.
Zero to sixty thoughts per second,
or was I worrying and planning all night,
dreading the day's inevitable disasters?

I force a breath,
another, slightly easier.
Eyes urged open;
a choice is made--to live!
Rise, flush water over body,
a prayer of gratitude.
Hesitate, then move quickly, proudly,
past the computer, to the garden!
Space to be, to feel--more life!

Breaking patterns now,
allowing moments of magic,
awake, watching, present,
a color, an invitation,
listening, trusting.

Today,
disaster is delightfully denied.

THE STEP *April 20, 2009*

This is your Life
what you came here to do.
Body shudders, mind rushes me away
from the voice.

This is it,
the object of your desperate pleas
and heartfelt prayers!
Urgency this time!

But I can't, not yet, not ever.
Stop terrifying me with impossible invitations
to the party I cannot attend.

Then one day
drops a seed,
small, but suddenly relentless.
And somehow, moving quickly,
past napping negativity,
past countless small and desperate hands
and megaphone mouths,
a small, shaky yet certain step
finds the Earth,
where roots sprout,
and angels fill the sky.

SCORCHED EARTH *July 5, 2009*

What if I loosened,
my carefully controlled grip?
What if I trusted my gut,
ceased to deny the dreaded backlog?

If I emoted, fully,
if the dam suddenly burst,
would the fury unleashed
prove the wisdom of restraint?

Or would violence be the inevitable consequence
of continued compaction?
If I let go, would I scorch the Earth,
or would the lava flow slow
and grief find bottom?

Would fear's suffocation
and denial's devils be purged,
replaced by divine spaciousness?

Shall I play it safe
and continue the culturally demanded constriction,
assuring my deadly descent?

Or feel, trust, dance,
unburden my beloved body,
and quite possibly,
be free.

NO ORDINARY MOMENTS *July 5, 2009*

Cycles and rhythms, yes,
but nature knows no repetition.
Every leaf and raindrop unique.

If life is boring,
what are you ignoring?

Let the child guide you to your belly,
to sniff meadow grass,
rub noses with grasshopper,
as your toes become moist.

Soften body--don't think!
Close your eyes and see,
open the sacred senses.

Nothing the same,
no ordinary moments.

FROG FEELINGS *August 7, 2009*

I'm not sure exactly
why frogs make me happy.
We may not even see eye to eye,
but what a joy to see one!

Alejandro, a Huichol Indian in Mexico,
told me, *La rana canta cuando viene la lluvia*
(frogs sing when the rains come).
How I love that song
as I love the rain!

They say that frogs are sensitive to human ways
and are disappearing.
Why do I hurt what I say I love?
Now, when I see a frog,
I am happy and sad.

DANCE IN THE DARK *September 5, 2009*

Dance, in the dark.
Never miss a song.
Every gaffe a gift.
Acceptance makes you strong.

Dance, with your courage,
though you may look a fool,
fall flat on your face,
for whom you need look cool?

Dance, laugh, pray,
with feelings that shout,
failure, loser, bad!
Breathe and cry throughout.

Dance with your deepest pain,
drawn it close to your breast.
No longer can they hurt you.
Welcome, invited guests.

TOO LATE?   *October 10, 2009*

What a beautiful planet
we are destroying.

No, Earth will save herself by shifting, purging,
removing many of us.

We suffocate,
cook and starve ourselves slowly,
pretend that water is a commodity,
fearfully cling to unessential lies and lives.

Take a breath.
Feel your body!
Listen, reconnect
with the bigger body Earth
and with the Everything.

See no other, and stop the madness.
End this mass suicide.
Let ego needs diminish and follow Nature's way.

I hope and pray
it is not too late.

BATTLE READY *October 20, 2009*

The inner ocean has calmed
as the outer storm approaches.

I am so blessed!
That dreaded, draining depression
and demonic moodiness
stabilized somewhat.
My castle fortified
in preparation for battle, or surrender.

The suffocating sadness and relentless fear
at long last dissolved
back into joy and gratitude,
leaving me here now,
trusting, loving, breathing, alive,
less afraid,
but still afraid.

COSMIC CRAYON *November 1, 2009*

Behold a splendid forest,
infinite shades of yellow, green and red.
From one cosmic color,
with a stroke of divine brush,
a rainbow from Beyond.

WHAT CONTROL? *December 7, 2009*

What, if anything,
do I control?
Thoughts, perhaps,
and therefore everything.
Including Earth changes?
Mayan, Hopi prophesies:
end of times,
beginning of times.
26,000 year cycle.

Predictable shift,
or are we responsible?
Have we helped create a new golden age,
or did we mess up?
Even if we work together--
which we are not, yet--
is it still too late?
Perhaps only divine magic
can save us now.
Or are salvation and survival inevitable?

Surrender control
to the One
who knows, controls everything,
yet allows us freedom and choice
to *be* the One
to control anything,
or nothing
or everything.

FEAR NOT *Dec 12, 2009*

What is real, what is true?
2012, we have a clue.

Mayan prophesies, crystallized wisdom,
yet no one knows what in truth may come.

Apocalyptic warnings, end of times,
or golden age, new paradigm?

From Kali Yoga dark and ailing Earth,
masculine balance, feminine rebirth.

Elders say, do not fear.
Be in the heart, the dawn is near.

BREATH OF THE MANTA RAY *December 18, 2009*

What does it say
about me and our world
that when I consider breathing
naturally, easily, deeply,
I become stressed and confused
and rely on my overused companions,
mind and intellect?
Why do I need read
a book on natural breathing?

Can I not learn to permit nature's prana
to caress my hardened heart?
If I allow the prana passage
below the chest-guards,
and enter, bowing, to belly's compactions,
can I not thaw the frozen fears?

Body, mind and spirit,
seemingly impossible task:
reuniting a feuding family,
all with interests of their own.

Invite breath as the bridge and balm.
Let diaphragm gently ebb and flow--
wings of the manta ray,
every breath a massage.

Normal is insane.
We hurl heavy-metal motorized machines
faster than most can throw a baseball.
Pave over everything,
then, on weekends, tired and worn,
follow this same pavement
back to nature.

Some suck bucket-sized
overpriced sugar water.
Some treat the wounded
in toxic, bacteria-breeding grounds called hospitals.
Some blow the tops off mountains,
and keep nature photos on their walls.
Some spill toxins in rivers,
then spend enormous time and money
filtering the toxins downstream--and send us the bill.
Some receive enormous subsidies
to pour pesticides on industrial crops,
and eat organic foods at home.

Some question all this,
and are called radical troublemakers,
trying to ruin such a good thing.

And yet others
see the perfection in even this,
always with eyes both here and beyond.

RELATIONSHIP *December 20, 2009*

A relationship ends,
and people offer that look,
"I'm so sorry it didn't work out."

Ah, but of course it did!
If I only knew the million primordial twists and turns
that led to this holy encounter,
be it a glance on the street,
a scowl--or smile--from a neighbor,
the life partner.

If only I recognized how perfect and adventurous,
a divorce as delirious and delicious as a honeymoon!
All perfect: taking this, giving that,
karma created, karma cleared,
Our relationship has ancient roots,
and is just getting started.

I may not act it, or show it, or even know it,
but how I love you!
and you!
and you!

THE TEACHER   *December 22, 2009*

It is always such a relief
to have my ignorance acknowledged.

One day, after class,
a student approaches me, hesitates,
then with bitter certainty,
"I just realized that you have no idea
what you are talking about!
In fact, I know as much as you!"

Halleluiah!
I taught one well.

ANGRY-LOVING MOTHER   *December 25, 2009*

We know something is wrong,
roaring and grumbling,
Mother Earth is terribly upset.
We wonder why,
yet know,
our guilt a clue.

We have ignored, taken Mother for granted,
assumed her love and patience
are stronger than her fury.
But our constant fighting and craving,
our love of toys,
has poisoned our home,
made Mother sick.

She may recover,
as she is much bigger and stronger than us.
And how she still loves us!
How this must cause her anguish,
to punish, even sacrifice,
some of her own children.
Know that she does so
all for good,
with love.

AWAKEN! *Dec 29, 09*

Though eyes blur and draw downward
and heart be heavy . . .

Awaken!

Though the world
draws you unconscious,
into its drunken dismay,
where even children lose their luster . . .

Awaken!

Shake and move, before
discs rust over
and seal prana's doorways . . .

Awaken!

from an unseen sunrise,
and just another day,
to a sunrise!
and this moment!

From wasteful worries and
mind's manic trap,
to delightful Presence,
eyes that shout--I see You!

How can you sleep,
locked in a closet full of karmic cobwebs,
when all round you,
an open invitation,
the flutter of angel wings.
Freedom beckons, invites you
into ecstatic meadows and mountains
of multihued magic and majesty.

Awaken

Keep not your lover waiting.

2010 *January 1, 2010*

2009, in many ways,
depressing decade,
following history's deadliest century.
Can hope be justified in 2010?

Yes!
Watch alchemy transform and
diminish the age of darkness,
iron to gold.
Not without chaos and upheaval,
shaking us from our discomfort zone,
lighting up every secret and illusion,
lining us up
to face one another:
Christian and Muslim,
Arab and Jew,
believers and non-believers,
Northern eagle and Southern condor.

How to prepare?
Ancients and prophets,
from every age, every language, every scripture:
Know thyself.
Love thy neighbor.
Be as a child.
Honor Mother Earth
and Father Sky.
Attach to nothing.
Fear nothing.
Love everything.

Nature Knows *June 8, 2010*

Flexibility and flow,
nature knows.
Seasons come,
seasons go.

Oh how we try,
never asking why,
regulate and control,
our nature denied.

Spring thaws snows,
rivers that flow.
Blossoms and buds,
vibrant greens aglow.

Leaf leans to the sun,
herd on the run.
Summer is born.
Marmots have fun!

Berries for bears,
as cool turns the air.
Furs thicken,
nests prepared.

Once again we meet,
frigid old friend we greet.
Slow and surrender,
into winter's retreat.

Body Spirit   *November 1, 2010*

Body trembles,
regretting past,
fretting future.

Breathe,
the purity of Presence.
Sense,
the One within,
who knows no fear,
celebrating past and creating future
from the Now.

CATASTROPHE OR ECSTASY? *November 5, 2010*

Armageddon? Apocalypse? End times?
End of world, or end of world as we know it?
Breakdown or breaththrough?
Deniers of Earth changes
as confused
as those declaring doomsday.

You are God --
how could God be doomed!?
Death or life?
Ending or beginning?
As always, both.

You are the creative source
consciously and courageously
here, on Earth, now.
Universal intelligence itself, naturally, beautifully
orchestrating the great turning,
The shift from duality to unity,
dimness and density,
to quickening light,
the great purification,
cycling from a well-worn age of numbed ignorance,
dumbed and darkened denial.

Fret not, fear not.
Ride the wave.
Create and cultivate
a new World Age.

RESURRECTION *December 25, 2010*

Blessings upon blessings!
From an age of war and frozen fear,
depression and darkened despair,
to chants of praise and gratitude.
To be here, now,
this most magnificent moment,
the resurgence of Mother Earth!

Welcome the return of saints and sages,
not judgment and punishment,
but liberation and celebration,
resurrect, renew and remind us:
Holy one, we have heard your cry in the night.
Peacemaker, your work did not go unnoticed.
Light worker, your faith has set you free.
Dear one, you have heard the warnings of dread and doom,
yet broken the prophesies,
the Now's power over prediction.

Feel the shift!
Delay not the celebration
by dreading days of judgment.
For you, embodied angel,
are revered, honored, loved.
The entire Universe
blesses and applauds you!

COURAGEOUS CONTEMPLATION *1/1/11*

Narcissistic navel gazing
and mental masturbation?
Or subversive self-awakening,
knowing the Universe?

Questions asked only by he
who has not stilled the mind
and ventured from head to heart.

Ever more are tasting
the sweetness of divine grace,
moving from thinking to feeling,
from robotic following and reacting,
to leading and living!

Growing numbers shifting
from cleverness and calculation
to wonder and amazement.
From strain and stress
to breathing and being.
From accepting a world gone mad
to sacred activism and settling for no less
than a heavenly humanity.

Stillness, presence, divine doing --
tools of the new Earth warrior.

NATURE PRAYER *February 2, 2011*

Divine Spirit,
may I be like your old growth cedar,
resilient, rooted in the Earth,
yet growing, reaching for the heavens.

May I be humble like the butterfly,
yet bold as the bear,
bright as the stars.

May my love be like the sun, always strong,
shining on friends and enemies alike.

May I be like the owl and crow,
wise and quick of thought.
Yet like the sloth and slug,
soft and slow.

May I be like the joyous, singing frog,
using my voice,
celebrating the transformation from shadow to light,
and like the thunderstorms and earthquakes,
healthfully expressing my emotions.

May I be like the rabbit and deer,
alert, quick, intuitive.
And like the stone,
solid, unshakeable.
Yet flowing, fluid like the stream,
ever moving towards the ocean of One.

May I be like the ant and bee,
working in community, utilizing my gifts,
yet resting, patient, and purring
like a curled, napping cat.

May I be like fire, enveloping all,
with my passion for peace and justice,
yet like the moon, a soft, soothing presence,
and like the darkness,
inviting all within to play with our shadows,
and like the soil,
creating a nurturing space of love and growth.

And may everything in this world
be also like beloved me,
beautifully and powerfully created,
an image and likeness of divine love.

EARTH DAY   *April 22, 2011*

It starts, perhaps, with a day,
then, moment by moment,
with yoga, tai chi, barefoot connections,
we meditate and chant,
ancient ways revisited.

We begin anew, today,
learning to listen, to honor, to pray.
We bow, forehead and fingers to Earth,
our tears nourishing soil and seed.

We remember our roots:
singing and dancing, healing and growing,
hearing our Mother's cries and calls
to come home, clean up after ourselves,
knowing that Mother still loves us.

Forgive me, Mother, for pain I have caused you.
Know too, that I have always loved *you*.

Unfiltered Feet *May 3, 2011*

The first steps, tender reminders
of my lost nature,
my civilized soles.
Then, step by step, stone by stone, skin to soil,
grounding, opening, releasing,
reconnecting with Mother Earth,
a surge of strength and satisfaction,
barefoot with my beloved,
kissing the Earth with every step,
I return to my roots.

WHO I AM *June 14, 2011*

Who am I?
Who am I?
Who am I?

I am everything
yet no thing,
empty.

I am the silence
at the source
of sound.

CEDAR WISDOM *June 25, 2011*

Ground, embrace, watch.
Ground--connect deeply with the Earth.
Embrace--without judgment, what is.
Watch--what happens within and around you.

As we trees do.
Watching humans come and go.
Watching life unfold.
Watching the changing Earth.
Stand tall and watch.

Do not be uprooted by the winds of life,
though one day you will fall.
When that day comes,
do not hold on--let go.
Fall easily, naturally,
with gratitude for your time on Earth.
Enjoy the fall!

Know that nothing dies,
all moving back into the great
and beautiful
cycle of life.

BE YOU *July 11, 2011*

Be true
to You
Not *you*--You!

If we only knew,
the path of the few.
Here is a clue:

Be more than do.
Not around pain but through,
with Spirit's view,
rejoice and renew.
Woo hoo!

MESSAGE TO THE DARK SIDE *July 15, 2011*

Forces of darkness, known by many names:
Illuminati, secret government, ruling elite, devil.
Whoever, wherever you are, I have a message:
Today, this minute, I declare immunity from your evil.
No longer can you scare, hurt, confuse or program me.

For far too long you have suffocated me with your schools,
controlled me with religious rules,
and convinced me of my powerlessness.
You have tried to take me out, and failed.

Although you are cowardly despots,
I resist and judge you not.
I have arisen from my sleepy, sheepy state.
I honor your ignorance and essential innocence,
as I welcome and embrace my own shadows,
validating both my own and your pitiful violations.

I stand here, open arms and heart,
awaiting, inviting you,
back into the light.

Back to hell?
Or join us on the new heaven on Earth?
What do you choose?

SACRED MASCULINE *July 20, 2011*

Men, it is time!
to redefine, recreate
healthy masculinity,
to show up, stand up, power up
and sometimes step down, soften,
balancing yin with yang.

The warrior follows the whisper of his own heart,
while the soldier follows orders.

This green man is fatherly, not dominant,
embodies peace--like Saint Francis,
connects with nature and Earth,
balancing left and right brain.

This spiritual warrior speaks out
about violent movies and war machines,
yet is comfortable with silence.
Before grabbing a beer, or turning on TV,
he feels what stirs within,
walks willingly into his shadows.

He connects with other men,
inviting them into their integrity,
back home to beloved body
to feel and heal.

He stops projecting his own missing father issues
on an absent or abusive God,
does not confuse injurious religion
with healthy spirituality.

He feels his freedom curtailed
when millions of brothers are jailed,

by a toxic, profit-run prison system.
This man exudes compassion and integrity,
speaks truth to power and injustices
of our "civilized" world
that divide and conquer
and harden the heart.

He confronts centuries of shame
and expresses healthy sexuality,
imperfectly yet fully relates to women,
honoring and celebrating the new and ancient feminine.

This man knows his worth beyond success and production,
knowing how to rest.
He grows with ritual,
drums and dances,
prays and plays,
speaks and listens,
fails and falls,
succeeds and celebrates.

This is the new man of the new paradigm,
shifting from wounded warrior
and distorted, depleted maleness,
moving from scared and scarred, to sacred masculine.
He knows his Christ-Buddha nature,
and becomes the new role model,
a man of great peace,
a man among men,
a beautiful man.

AGING GRACE *July 23, 2011*

Are we elderly
or elders?

Does the world look down on us
or up to us?
Does the way we live our life
have anything to do with this?

Are we already dead,
spiritless bodies clutching harsh judgments
of what could have been?
Or timeless souls,
laughing at our follies,
celebrating and applauding our humanity?

Are we bitter about barely walking,
or joyfully rocking!

Are we
growing old without growth,
aging without grace?
Or watching, listening,
always learning,
teaching by being?

Does our presence darken and depress a place,
or brighten and create sacred space?

Do we wall off our youth,
even as we grow dependent on them,
judging and projecting our embittered failures?
Or welcome and encourage them to show us a new way?

Do we have both feet in the grave,
or one foot in each world,
Earth and Spirit,
like wise, old growth trees,
touching heaven, rooting deeply,
drawing from Earth experience,
our last breath a blessing.

Pain Poems, Passion Poems *August 1, 2011*

Less pain--less poems.
Was my pen only moved and motivated by
suffering and struggle?
Do I only write and pray when in need?
Hungry heart's longing for my Beloved
bent my knees,
frenzied, frantic journalings.

Has my path now become so sated
with pleasure and play,
life and love,
community and celebration?!
From beggar's pleas and desperate scribbles
to delight and gratitude in every breath.
Prayers are answered!

Why write to the Friend
who hears my every thought--before I think it!
who whispers in my ear--before I ask!
Why search for the One
who lives so close in my heart.

QUICK ORDER FORM

Website Orders: Please go to www.Holmanhealthconnections.com
and follow the book & CD order links.

Telephone Orders: Call 425-303-8150.
Have credit card ready (or leave message and we will call you back soon).

Postal Orders: Send check to
Holman Health Connections
1917 Rockefeller Ave.,
Everett, WA 98201 USA

Name: _____

Address: _____State: _____ Zip: _____

Country / Phone: _____

Email (to receive Roy's monthly Enewsletter): _____

Please send me these items, knowing
I may return them for a full refund within 30 days.

Poems from the Passionate Heart _____ (quantity) @ $12.95 = _____

Healing Self, Healing Earth (book) _____ @ $15.95 each = _____

Meditation CD: (5 meditations) _____ @ $12.95 each = _____

Shipping: $4.00 for first book or CD,
and $2.00 for each additional: _____

International: $8.00 for first book or CD,
and $4.00 each additional: _____

Sales Tax: WA state residents please add approximate sales tax: _____

Total enclosed:

_____

THANK YOU!

Also by Roy Holman

1. "Healing Self, Healing Earth:
Awakening Presence, Power, and Passion"
Copyright © 2010 by Roy Holman
Softcover Edition ISBN 978-0-615-29882-5
$15.95

2. Meditation CD
Includes five meditations:
1. Breath and Being
2. Manifestation Meditation
3. Chakra Meditation
4. Sleepytime Meditation
5. Meditative flute (background flute by Stef Frenzl)
$12.95

Feedback on Roy's poems, other books and classes

• *What a gift these poems are for anyone who reads them!* Mari Avedano

• *I have just come across your superb poem, "Eating My Way To God." I haven't laughed at myself so hard in years! You are totally right. What am I playing at with all this guilt? I eat two sunflower seeds which have been "exposed to heat" and my day is ruined!!!!!!!! Thank you. You have set me free. 'Tis better to eat pizza with friends that to eat sprouts alone!* Haley, Dublin, Ireland

• *This is the most 'real' and grounded approach to ancient wisdom I have ever read.* Jennifer Elais, Australia (about Healing Self, Healing Earth)

• *Thank you for your kindness. I want you to know that your class touches more than just the muscles; it touches the soul.* Rhonda, Everett, Washington

• *Your poems resonate with me; certainly I have been through enough failed relationships and lost loves--the most important of those being the one with myself. Hopefully it is not too late to resurrect that one!* Catherine, Everett, Washington

• *The yoga classes are awesome, but what I love the best about class is the reminder of who I really am, a spiritual being on this amazing earthly journey. Thanks for all the gentle reminders to do the "inner" work.* Elaine, Everett, Washington

• *Roy is a gifted wounded healer who gives voice to the pain within us all and offers hope and courage to transcend it.* Donna Vande Kieft, hospice chaplain, seeker of truth and transformation